Silver Educational Publishing
Published by Silver 8 Production LLC

ISBN 0-9719996-8-6

Other Titles Available From SILVER EDUCATIONAL PUBLISHING (SEPBOOKS.COM)

Anatomy and Physiology Study Guide: Key Review Questions and Answers with Explanations (Volume 1)

Anatomy and Physiology Study Guide: Key Review Questions and Answers with Explanations (Volume 2)

Key Facts for Anatomy and Physiology

Microbiology Study Guide: Key Review Questions and Answers

Spinal Anatomy Study Guide: Key Review Questions and Answers

CONTENTS

The Cell Cytoplasm
Answers are in the back.

1. Which is not true of the eukaryotic cell?
   a. These cells are generally smaller than prokaryotic cells.
   b. Organelles are found in the cytoplasm.
   c. Has a nuclear envelope
   d. The nucleus is separated from the rest of the organelles in the cytoplasm.

2. Which of the following is a component of the cytoplasm?
   a. cell inclusions
   b. organelles
   c. cytosol
   d. all of the above

3. The _______ consists of all the cellular components found between the nucleus and the plasma membrane.
   a. cell inclusion
   b. cytoplasm
   c. glycolipid
   d. extra-cellular substance

4. The plasma membrane is mainly composed of proteins and lipids.
   a. true
   b. false

5. 75% of all lipids in the plasma membrane are ________.
   a. glycolipids
   b. cholesterol
   c. phospholipids
   d. testosterone

6. Which separates the cytoplasm form the extracellular surroundings?
   a. cell membrane
   b. glycolipid
   c. organelle
   d. cytosol

7. Which of the following is not a component of the cell membrane (plasmalemma)?

a. glycolipid
b. cholesterol
c. glycoprotein
d. cytosol

Cell Organelles

8. Cellular respiration occurs in the _________.

a. mitochondria
b. lysosomes
c. golgi appartus
d. nucleus

9. Lysosomes work best at a(n) ________ pH; they are formed in the ________.

a. acidic, mitochondria
b. acidic, golgi complex
c. basic, mitochondria
d. basic, golgi complex

10. Which of the following packages and delivers proteins to the plasma membrane and to lysosomes?

a. mitochondria
b. nucleus
c. ribosome
d. golgi complex

11. Medial, Trans and Cis cisterns are located in the ________.

a. golgi complex
b. ribosome
c. nucleus
d. mitochondria

12. The largest structure of the eukaryotic cell is the ________.

a. ribosome
b. endoplasmic reticulum
c. mitochondria

d. nucleus

13. Protein synthesis occurs in the ________, which is made in the ________.

a. lysosome, nucleus
b. mitochondria, nucleolus
c. ribosome, smooth ER
d. ribosome, nucleolus

14. Which of the following organelles is responsible for producing ATP and hence, is called the powerhouse of the cell?

a. nucleus
b. ribosome
c. mitochondria
d. lysosome

15. Which of the following is a function of the cytoskeleton?

a. cell movement
b. shape cells
c. support cells
d. all of the above

16. Microtubules, microfilaments, and intermediate filaments are ________ that make up the ________.

a. fats, cytoskeleton
b. proteins, cytoskeleton
c. fats, ER
d. proteins, ER

17. The cytoskeleton is located in the cytoplasm; it allows for cell movement and support of organelles.

a. true
b. false

18. Lipid and carbohydrate synthesis occur in the ________.

a. ribosome
b. endoplasmic reticulum
c. nucleolus

d. cytoskeleton

19. Which of the following is not true of agranular ER?
    a. has a network of polyribosomes
    b. detoxifies carcinogens in our body
    c. place of steroid and phospholipid production
    d. place of fatty acid synthesis

20. Intracellular digestion occurs at the ________.
    a. ribosome
    b. lysosome
    c. golgi apparatus
    d. nucleus

21. Digestion of an extracellular substance by a lysosome is called ________.
    a. autophagy
    b. heterophagy
    c. cellular respiration
    d. autolysis

22. Cilia and flagella contain ________ pairs of ________.
    a. 8, intermediate filiaments
    b. 8, microfilaments
    c. 9, microtubules
    d. 4, microtubules

23. Which of the following is composed of nine clusters of microtubule triplets found in a round pattern within the centrosome?
    a. cilia
    b. flagella
    c. centriole
    d. cell inclusion

24. All of the following are cell inclusions except?
    a. triglycerides
    b. glycogen
    c. melanin

d. lysosome

25. Lysosomes break down _________.
    a. proteins
    b. nucleic acid
    c. carbohydrates
    d. all of the above

26. Which of the following is composed of microtubules?
    a. cilia and flagella
    b. mitotic spindle
    c. mitotic spindle
    d. all of the above

27. Regular ribosomes attach to the ER and, free ribosomes do not attach to any organelles.
    a. true
    b. false

28. ATP is produced in the ________,which have interior foldings called ________.
    a. golgi complex, cisterns
    b. nucleus, cisterns
    c. mitochondria, cristae
    d. centrosomes, centrioles

29. Which of the following organelles is the largest and stores genes?
    a. ribosome
    b. nucleus
    c. lysosome
    d. golgi complex

Mitosis and Meiosis

30. Which is the correct progressive order of events in the cell cycle?
    a. G_1 phase, S phase, G_2 phase, mitosis, cytokinesis
    b. mitosis, S phase, cytokinesis, G_1 phase, G_2 phase
    c. S phase, G_1 phase, G_2 phase, mitosis, cytokinesis

d. mitosis, cytokinesis, G_1 phase, S phase, G_2 phase

31. There are _______ pairs of chromosomes that are sex chromosomes called _______.

a. 23, autosomes
b. 23, somatic cells
c. 22, autosomes
d. 22, centrioles

32. Which of the following is not a stage of mitosis that consists of the majority of the time of the cell cycle?

a. interphase
b. metaphase
c. anaphase
d. prophase

33. Which of the following phases of meiosis are dissimilar to the corresponding phase of mitosis?

a. anaphase I
b. metaphase II
c. prophase II
d. telophase II

34. Mitosis I is referred to as the _________ and meiosis II is called the ________ phase.

a. equatorial division phase, reduction division
b. reduction division phase, equatorial division

35. The synthesis of eggs and sperm is accomplished in _________ and ______ is used for the production of somatic cells or cells of the body.

a. meiosis, mitosis
b. mitosis, meiosis
c. mitosis, meiosis II
d. meiosis, meiosis II

36. DNA replication occurs during _________ of meiosis I and mitosis.

a. prophase
b. telophase

c. anaphase
d. interphase

37. Which of the following stages is divided into G_1 phase, S phase, and G_2 phase?
a. anaphase
b. prophase
c. interphase
d. telophase

38. DNA synthesis and replication occur during the ________ phase of ________
a. S, interphase
b. S, prophase
c. G_1, interphase
d. G_2, telophase

39. RNA synthesis occurs in the G_1 phase of interphase.
a. true
b. false

40. The cleavage furrow can be first observed in ________ of meiosis and mitosis.
a. metaphase
b. interphase
c. anaphase
d. telophase

41. Mitosis and cytokinesis consists of _______ hours in the cell cycle.
a. 5-6
b. 4-5
c. 1-2
d. 23

42. The final stage of mitosis is referred to as:
a. interphase
b. telophase
c. anaphase

d. metaphase

43. Chromosomes and centromeres line up in the center of the cell in _________ of mitosis.

a. interphase
b. metaphase
c. telophase
d. anaphase

44. 90 % of the cell cycle accounts for __________.

a. interphase
b. metaphase
c. mitosis
d. cytokinesis

45. Cell division that results in the synthesis of sperm and eggs is called ________.

a. mitosis
b. meiosis

46. Which of the following is a function of the lysosome?

a. bacteria digestion
b. autolysis
c. autophagy
d. all of the above

Epithelial Tissue

47. Which is a basic type of connective tissue in the body?

a. nervous
b. epithelial
c. muscular
d. connective
e. all of the above

48. Which type of connective tissue consists of polyhedral cells with a tiny amount of intercellular substance?

a. connective

b. epithelial
c. nervous
d. muscular

49. Epithelia lining the skin is primarily derived from
a. ectoderm
b. endoderm
c. mesoderm
d. all of the above

Matching:

50. The lining of respiratory and digestive tracts are mainly derived from _________.	a. ectoderm
51. The endothelial lining of blood vessels is derived from _________.	b. mesoderm
52. The epithelium lining the nose, skin and anus are derived from ________.	c. squamous
53. Flattened nuclei are specifically found in ________ cells.	d. endoderm

54. Which of the following is a shape of epithelial cell nuclei?
a. spherical
b. elongated
c. elliptic
d. all of the above

55. Cuboidal cells have flattened nuclei.
a. true
b. false

Cuboidal cells have spherical nuclei. The correct answer is B.

56. Basal lamina is found around which of the following?
a. adipose tissue
b. muscle and epithelial tissue
c. Schwann cells

d. all of the above

57. The basement lamina is a component of the ________.
    a. connective tissue
    b. epithelium
    c. basement membrane
    d. apical surface

58. Which of the following connects the epithelium with the connective tissue?
    a. basement membrane
    b. apical surface
    c. polyhedral cells
    d. contractile cells

59. All of the following are components of the basal lamina except:
    a. laminin
    b. proteoglycan
    c. collagen
    d. connective tissue

60. ________ is not a part of the basal lamina.
    a. lamina densa
    b. laminae lucidae
    c. epithelium
    d. laminae rarae

61. Which type of basement membrane is located in the kidney glomerulus and alveoli of the lung?
    a. fusion of two basal laminae
    b. basal lamina and reticular lamina

62. Which type of basement membrane is the most common type found in the body?
    a. fusion of two basal laminae
    b. basal lamina and reticular lamina

63. Which is a function of intercellular junctions in epithelial tissue?

a. serve as a seal between cells
b. promote cell aggregation
c. help in the communication and cohesion between cells
d. all of the above

64. Anchoring junctions are common in which of the following locations?
a. outer layer of skin
b. muscle tissue of heart
c. neck of uterus
d. epithelial lining of GI tract
e. all of the above

65. Zonula occludens is referred to as a
a. tight junction
b. desmosome
c. hemidesmosome
d. macula adherens

66. Which is a type of communicating junction that forms little tunnel-like structures known as connexons?
a. desmosome
b. zona occludens
c. hemidesmosome
d. gap junction

67. __________ is located in the apex of the cell.
a. zona occludens
b. gap junction
c. hemidesmosome
d. desmosome

68. All of the following are classified as adhering junctions except:
a. desmosomes
b. zonulae occludentes
c. hemidesmosomes
d. zonulae adherentes

69. Which of the following is not a type of simple epithelium?

a. glandular
b. columnar
c. cuboidal
d. squamous

70. The epidermis is characterized by which type of epithelium?
a. transitional
b. glandular
c. stratified squamous keratinized
d. stratified squamous nonkeratinized

71. Which is not true of stereocilia?
a. they are long and motile
b. they are long and nonmotile
c. there are longer branched microvilli
d. they increase surface area of the cell

72. Which is not true of the microvilli?
a. It is an extension of the cytoplasm.
b. It is covered by the plasma membrane.
c. Microvilli help in increasing absorption to the cell.
d. Microvilli are usually found at the bottom of the cell.

73. Which of the following grows from a basal body?
a. microvilli
b. cilia
c. flagella
d. stereocilia

74. Which type of epithelium consists of more than one layer of cells?
a. simple
b. simple cuboidal
c. stratified
d. simple columnar

75. Stratified epithelium is classified:
a. by the cell shape of its superficial layer
b. by the cell shape of its most inferior layer

c. by the number of cells it contains
d. under a type of simple epithelium

76. Which type of cell serves as the covering for the ovary?
    a. simple squamous
    b. stratified squamous keratinized
    c. simple cuboidal
    d. simple columnar

77. All of the following are lined by transitional epithelium except:
    a. urinary bladder
    b. ureter
    c. renal calyces
    d. conjunctiva

78. Which type of epithelium lines the intestines and gallbladder?
    a. simple cuboidal
    b. transitional
    c. simple squamous
    d. stratified columnar

79. Lining of blood vessels and the mesothelium is composed of:
    a. simplc cuboidal
    b. simple squamous
    c. stratified columnar
    d. transitional

80. The basal lamina connects the lamina propria and the epithelial tissues.
    a. true
    b. false

81. Which of the following is part of the connective tissue and helps support the epithelial and not part of the basement membrane?
    a. basal lamina
    b. reticular lamina
    c. connexon
    d. lamina propria

82. Epithelium is divided into two types: covering epithelia and glandular epithelia.

a. true
b. false

83. Glands form from covering epithelium.

a. true
b. false

84. The most superficial layer of the epidermis is the __________.

a. dermal papilla
b. stratum lucidum
c. stratum corneum
d. stratum basale

85. The epidermis is derived from the

a. ectoderm
b. mesoderm
c. endoderm
d. all of the above

86. Approximately 90% of epidermal cells are made of

a. Merkel cells
b. Langerhans cells
c. keratinocytes
d. melanocytes

87. Which of the following layers is directly superior to the dermis?

a. stratum basale
b. stratum lucidum
c. stratum granulosum
d. stratum corneum

88. The ________ is located exclusively in the stratum basale; it has a function in the sense of touch.

a. Langerhans cell
b. Merkel cell
c. keratinocyte

d. melanocyte

89. The epidermis consists of which of the following cells?
    a. keratinocytes
    b. melanocytes
    c. Langerhans cell
    d. Merkel cell
    e. all of the above

90. The stratum basale has ________ and ________ cells.
    a. squamous, cuboidal
    b. columnar, squamous
    c. squamous, transitional
    d. columnar, cuboidal

91. Keratinocytes are produced by stem cells predominately in the
    a. stratum basale
    b. stratum spinsoum
    c. stratum lucidum
    d. stratum granulosum

92. The stratum lucidum is most apparent in
    a. palms of the hands and soles of the feet
    b. back of the neck
    c. lumbar area
    d. skull

93. Which of the following is not true about pseudostratified epithelium?
    a. it has one layer of cells
    b. all of its cells adhere to the basal lamina
    c. it is multi-layered
    d. it lines the trachea and bronchi

94. Which type of gland is ductless and secretes its products into extracellular fluid?
    a. endocrine glands
    b. exocrine glands
    c. simple glands

d. multicellular glands

95. __________ is a type of gland that has ducts; they maintain their connection to the epithelial surface.
   a. endocrine
   b. exocrine
   c. holocrine
   d. merocrine

96. Which type of epithelium allows for distention or stretching and is located in the lining for the urinary bladder?
   a. stratified squamous
   b. transitional
   c. stratified cuboidal
   d. simple squamous

97. Goblet cells are found in the small intestine and the repiratory tract.
   a. true
   b. false

98. Which of the following is a secretion of an exocrine gland?
   a. oil and wax
   b. perspiration
   c. mucus
   d. digestive enzymes
   e. all of the above

99. All of the following are types of endocrine glands except:
   a. sweat gland
   b. adrenal gland
   c. thyroid gland
   d. pituitary

100. If glands that are formed do not touch the surface epithelium, they are called __________ glands.
   a. exocrine
   b. endocrine

101. Which of the following is not a type of cellular organization for a simple gland that is classified exocrine?

a. coiled tubular
b. tubular
c. branched acinar
d. tubuloacinar

102. _________ is a type of exocrine gland, which has ducts that branch repeatedly.

a. compound gland
b. simple gland
c. goblet cell
d. all of the above

103. _________ is a type of exocrine gland, which has one unbranched duct.

a. simple gland
b. compound gland
c. compound acinar
d. compound tubuloacinar

104. Which of the following is a secretion of the endocrine gland?

a. wax
b. oil
c. mucus
d. hormone

105. Compound glands are types of exocrine glands that can be classified as __________.

a. tubular
b. tubuloacinar
c. acinar
d. all of the above

106. Epithelial cells in the intestines replace at a rate of 2-5 days by the process of mitosis.

a. true
b. false

107. Which type of gland uses exocytosis to get rid of its secretions?
   a. holocrine
   b. merocrine
   c. apocrine
   d. all of the above

108. Which of the following is a functional classification of an exocrine gland?
   a. holocrine
   b. apocrine
   c. merocrine
   d. all of the above

109. Protection is the general function of stratified epithelium.
   a. true
   b. false

110. Sweat glands are lined by __________ epithelia.
   a. transitional
   b. stratified cuboidal
   c. stratified columnar
   d. simple squamous

Matching:

111. Lining of wet cavities such as the esophagus and mouth	a. stratified columnar
112. Lines the ocular conjuctiva	b. simple cuboidal
113. Covers the ovary and thyroid. It has a function of secretion.	c. stratified squamous non keratinized
114. Function of distensibility and lines renal calyces	d. pseudostratified columnar
115. Lines the trachea, its nucleus is at different levels and not all of its cells touch the surface	e. transitional

116. Which of the following is false regarding Goblet cells?

a. This is a unicellular gland.
b. They are found in the epithelial lining of the urinary and reproductive systems.
c. They produce mucus.
d. They are classified as multicellular glands.

117. All of the following are types of simple epithelium except:

a. transitional
b. columnar
c. squamous
d. cuboidal

118. Which of the following lines the respiratory tract?

a. simple squamous
b. ciliated simple columnar
c. transitional
d. simple cuboidal

119. Secretory products are released into the bloodstream by _________ glands, and secretory products are released into ducts by _________ glands.

a. exocrine, endocrine
b. endocrine, exocrine

Connective Tissue

120. Connective tissue primarily develops from the ________, which is the _________ layer of the embryo.

a. endoderm, middle
b. mesoderm, outer
c. mesoderm, middle
d. ectoderm, outer

121. Extracellular matrix, which is the main component of connective tissue, is composed of:

a. ground substance
b. protein fibers
c. tissue fluid

d. all of the above

122. Which of the following is a type of connective tissue?
a. bone
b. areolar tissue
c. cartilage
d. all of the above

123. Mesenchymal cells produce mesenchyme, which is used in the making of all types of connective tissue.
a. true
b. false

124. _________ is used by the body to fill the spaces between connective tissue; it also acts a natural lubricate and barrier to foreign matter in the body.
a. mesenchyme
b. mesenchymal cells
c. ground substance
d. antibodies

125. Ground substance is composed of:
a. glycoprotein
b. proteoglycans
c. glycoaminoglycans
d. all of the above

126. A proteoglycan molecule is not made of a _________.
a. protein core
b. three-dimensional structure
c. glycosaminoglycan
d. macrophage

127. Immature cells in cartilage are called ________ and in bone _________.
a. chondroblasts, osteoblasts
b. chondroblasts, osteocytes
c. chondryocytes, osteoblasts

d. chondrocytes, osteocytes

128. _________ is a type of glycoaminoglycan found mostly in hyaline and elastic cartilages; it is jelly-like and provides support.

a. dermatan sulfate
b. chondroitin sulfate
c. collagen

129. Elastic fibers are located in the ________.

a. lungs
b. blood vessels
c. skin
d. all of the above

130. Which is not a type of connective tissue fiber?

a. reticular
b. elastic
c. collagen
d. merocrine

131. Reticular fibers are formed from __________, which is the most prevalent protein in the body.

a. collagen
b. elastin
c. laminin
d. all of the above

132. Which type of collagen is located mainly in hyaline and elastic cartilage where only thin fibrils are produced?

a. collagen type I
b. collagen type II
c. collagen type III
d. collagen type IV

133. Reticular fibers are composed mainly in collagen __________.

a. type I
b. type II
c. type III

d. type IV

134. Collagen is found in which of the following structures?
a. fibrous cartilage
b. ligaments
c. tendons and dermis
d. all of the above

135. Which of the following aids in the adhesion of chondrocytes to type II collagen?
a. fibronectin
b. laminin
c. chondronectin
d. all of the above

136. Which of the following types of collagen are most abundant in the body?
a. type I
b. type II
c. type III
d. type IV

137. Collage Type II is synthesized at which location?
a. fibroblast
b. chondroblast
c. osteoblast
d. Schwann cell

138. Collagen Type II is found usually in elastic cartilage and ________.
a. bone
b. smooth muscle
c. muscle basal laminae
d. hyaline cartilage

139. Collagen Type III is has a tissue distribution of all of the following except:
a. hyaline cartilage
b. smooth muscle

c. endoneurium
d. spleen

140. Which type of collagen is located around organs like the uterus and liver?
a. Type IV
b. Type III
c. Type II
d. Type V

141. Which of the following consists of linear polysaccharides with hexosamine and uronic acid?
a. structural glycoproteins
b. glycosaminoglycans

142. Hydroxyproline and hydroxylysine are amino acids that compose collagen.
a. true
b. false

143. Which of the following is an amino acid that is an ingredient of collagen?
a. proline
b. hydroxyproline
c. glycine
d. all of the above

144. Which of the following is most abundant in the elastic fiber system?
a. elaunin fibers
b. oxytalan fibers
c. elastic fibers
d. all of the above

145. Which of the following is directly responsible for the elasticity of the elastic fiber system?
a. elaunin fibers
b. oxytalan fibers
c. antibodies

d. elastic fibers

146. ________ is developed first in the development of the elastic fiber system.

a. elastic fiber
b. elaunin fiber
c. oxytalan fiber
d. all of the above

147. Which is the correct order of development of the elastic fiber system?

a. oxytalan fibers, elaunin fibers, elastic fibers
b. elastic fibers, oxytalan fibers, elaunin fibers
c. elastic fibers, elaunin fibers, oxytalan fibers
d. elaunin fibers, oxytalan fibers, elastic fibers

148. The production of antibodies is a responsibility of the ________.

a. fibroblast
b. osteoblast
c. plasma cell
d. eosinophilic leukocyte

149. Which of the following is most commonly found in connective tissue?

a. mast cell
b. fibroblast
c. plasma cell
d. monocyte

150. _________ produces fibers and ground substance, which contributes greatly to the structural function.

a. fibroblast
b. mast cell
c. adipose cell
d. lymphocyte

151. Which of the following is responsible for the making of collagen, elastic fiber, glycoproteins and glycoaminoglycans?

a. lymphocyte
b. monocyte

c. fibroblast
d. adipose cell

152. The mononuclear phagocyte system consists of _________ dispersed through out most organs of the body.
a. fibroblasts
b. macrophages
c. mast cells
d. adipose cells

153. Which of the following are considered macrophages?
a. osteoclasts
b. Kupffer cells in liver
c. microglial cells
d. all of the above

154. The most numerous types of cells present are macrophages and fibroblasts in __________ or areolar tissue.
a. loose connective tissue
b. dense connective tissue

155. Plasma cells are found in tissue inflammation, and in places of the body where bacteria can be found in high numbers. __________ are produced by these cells in response to antigens.
a. mast cells
b. antibodies
c. lymphocyte
d. adipose cell

156. Which of the following are usually found only in pathological conditions?
a. epitheloid cells
b. multinuclear giant cells
c. macrophages

157. All of the following are functions of the macrophage except:
a. phagocytosis
b. digestion

c. activation of immune system
d. cell-mediated resistance
e. production of ground substance

158. Monocytes mature in connective tissue where they become macrophages.
a. true
b. false

159. The _________ is a dilator of blood vessels during inflammation; its main function is to store chemicals involved with inflammation.
a. mast cell
b. fibroblast
c. macrophage
d. hyaluronic acid

160. Histamine is produced by which of the following?
a. fibroblast
b. macrophage
c. mast cell
d. fibrils

161. Which of the following is a type of areolar connective tissue?
a. collagen fibers
b. elastic fibers
c. reticular fibers
d. all of the above

162. Most connective tissue is derived from _________.
a. ectoderm
b. endoderm
c. mesenchyme
d. none of the above

163. Plasma cells develop from which of the following cells?
a. fibroblast
b. macrophage
c. B lymphocyte

d. dermatan sulfate

164. Which of the following helps to maintain the shape of the eyeball?
a. chondroitin sulfate
b. macrophage
c. dermatan sulfate
d. hyaluronic acid

165. Which of the following is not a type of dense connective tissue?
a. regular connective tissue
b. irregular connective tissue
c. elastic connective tissue
d. adipose tissue

166. Which of the following is not a type of loose connective tissue?
a. dense regular connective tissue
b. adipose tissue
c. reticular connective tissue
d. areolar connective tissue

167. _________ is somewhat fragile, very flexible and not too resistant to stress.
a. areolar connective tissue
b. dense irregular tissue
c. dense regular tissue
d. all of the above

168. Adipose tissue consists of brown fat mostly found in _______ and brown fat predominately occurring in ________.
a. infants, adults
b. adults, infants

169. Which is a type of mucous tissue that is made of ground substance and a larger part, hyaluronic acid?
a. macrophage
b. plasma cell
c. Wharton's jelly
d. non-embyronic connective tissue

170. All of the following are true regarding dense connective tissue except:

a. It is more resistant to stress as compared to loose connective tissue.
b. It consists mainly of collagen.
c. It is less flexible than loose connective tissue.
d. It is the most abundant type of connective tissue in the body.

171. Reticular cell is also known as a type of fibroblast.

a. true
b. false

172. Multilocular tissue or __________ adipose tissue is known to have large quantities of mitochondria.

a. brown
b. white
c. yellow
d. common

173. Adipocytes store __________, which is a major energy reserve.

a. protein
b. triglycerides
c. chondrocytes
d. dermatan sulfate

174. Which of the following is a function of connective tissue?

a. storage and support
b. transport
c. defense and repair
d. all of the above

175. Elastic fibers are abundant in the lungs, skin and blood vessels.

a. true
b. false

176. Unilocular adipose cells are _________ in adipose tissue.

a. spherical
b. polyhedral

177. Dense connective tissue has more cells than loose connective tissue.

However, dense connective tissue has a high proportion of collagen fibers.

a. true

b. false

Although both types of connective tissue have the same cells, there are more cells in loose connective tissue like fibroblasts, macrophages etc. The correct answer is B.

178. Which of the following types of connective tissue are arranged in a definite pattern in response to traction forces in one direction?

a. dense irregular connective tissue

b. dense regular connective tissue

179. Which of the following are directly or indirectly derived from a mesenchymal cell?

a. fibroblast

b. chondroblast

c. osteoblast

d. all of the above

180. The collagen of loose connective tissue is renewed at a faster pace than the collagen of dense regular connective tissue.

a. true

b. false

181. Which is the primary cell involved in connective tissue repair?

a. macrophage

b. histiocyte

c. fibroblast

d. plasma cell

182. Lymphocytes and macrophages predominate in the chronic stage of inflammation.

a. true

b. false

183. All of the following are colors of unilocular adipose tissue except:

a. yellow

b. white

c. dark yellow
d. brown

184. Which of the following is the color of multiocular adipose tissue?
a. brown
b. dark yellow
c. yellow
d. white

185. All of the following are true statements except:
a. Multiocular adipose tissue cells are larger than unilocular tissue.
b. Multiocular adipose tissue has a large quantity of mitochondria.
c. There is more white fat in adults than brown fat.
d. Uniocular adipose tissue has cells that have one large, central droplet of fat in its cytoplasm.

186. Which of the following can make fatty acids form glucose?
a. mast cell
b. reticular cell
c. adipose cell
d. all of the above

187. Which type of adipose tissue has fat droplets of various sizes in its cytoplasm?
a. multiocular tissue cells
b. uniociular tissue cells

188. Which of the following is false pertaining to uniocular adipose cells?
a. eccentric nucleus
b. each cell has multiple fat droplets without one large, central droplet
c. enormous amount of mitochondria
d. it is highly vascularized

189. Too much fat buildup in unilocular tissue is called ___________ obesity.
a. hyperplastic
b. hypertrophic

190. Uniocular adipose tissue is __________ innervated by the sympathetic division of the automonic nervous system; multiocular adipose tissue is __________ innervated by the sympathetic division.

a. indirectly, directly
b. directly, indirectly

191. An rise in the number of adipocytes will cause __________ .

a. hypertrophic obesity
b. hyperplastic obesity
c. starvation
d. scurvy

192. Which of the following is a function of cartilage?

a. aids in the develpoment of bone
b. provides a sliding area for joints
c. supports soft tissue
d. all of the above

193. ________ contains mostly type II collagen fibers; it is labeled the most common type of cartilage.

a. fibrocartilage
b. elastic cartilage
c. hyaline cartilage
d. none of the above

194. Cartilage contains cells called ________, which produce the extracellular matrix.

a. perichondrium
b. chondrocytes
c. mucous tissue
d. leukoctyes

195. Fibrocartilage contains type I collagen fibers; it is found in parts of the body that undergo great stress.

a. true
b. false

196. Which of the following is true pertaining to cartliage?

a. It is highly vascularized.
b. Cartilage has many nerves.
c. Lymphatic vessels are in cartilage.
d. hyaline cartilage is located in the larynx and nose.

197. Which of the following types of cartilage are avascular?
a. hyaline
b. elastic
c. fibrocartilage
d. all of the above

198. Fibrocartilage is found in all of the following places except:
a. intervertebral discs
b. symphysis pubis
c. the walls of respiratory passages such as the larynx and bronchi
d. menisci

199. _________ is derived from the notochord, and it is situated in a viscous substance of type II collagen fibrils and hyaluronic acid; it is found in the center of the intervertebral disc.
a. hyaline cartilage
b. nucleus pulposus
c. annulus fibrosus
d. elastic cartilage

200. The mature cartilage cell is called the __________, and the external surface of cartilage is enclosed by a layer of dense irregular connective tissue called the __________.
a. chondrocyte, perichondrium
b. chondroblast, perichondrium
c. chondrocyte, epiphyseal plate
d. chodroblast, epiphyseal plate

201. Cartilage expands from within is a type of ___________ growth.
a. appositional
b. interstitial

202. Which of the following is not surrounded by a perichondrium?
- a. elastic cartilage
- b. hyaline cartilage
- c. fibrocartilage
- d. all of the above have a perichondrium

203. Elastic cartilage can be located in all of the following locations except:
- a. external auditory canal
- b. auricle of ear
- c. epiglottis
- d. annulus fibrosus

204. Rows of chondrocytes are separated mostly by coarse collagen type I fibers, which is observed in ___________.
- a. fibrocartilage
- b. hyaline cartilage
- c. elastic cartilage
- d. perichondrium

205. Which is not true of the perichondrium?
- a. It composed of dense connective tissue.
- b. It holds the vascular supply for avascular cartilage.
- c. Articular cartilage has a perichondrium.
- d. Hyaline and elastic cartilage has perichondrium.

206. Hyaline cartilage is used as a temporary skeleton in fetal development; it will eventually become bone.
- a. true
- b. false

207. Which of the following is a mature cell that aids in the maintenance of the bone matrix?
- a. osteoblast
- b. osteocyte
- c. fibrocartilage
- d. hyaline cartilage

208. Which of the following is an external layer of bone that has osteogenic

cells?

a. endosteum
b. canaliculi
c. periosteum
d. all of the above

209. ________ does not have the ability of mitosis and is important in the making of the bone matrix.

a. osteoclast
b. osteocyte
c. osteoprogenitor cells
d. osteoblast

210. Which of the following is a component of the bone matrix?

a. glycoproteins
b. proteoglycans
c. type I collagen fibers
d. all of the above

211. When the osteoblast is surrounded by bone matrix, it then becomes an __________.

a. osteocyte
b. osteoclast
c. osteoprogenitor cell
d. elastic fiber

212. _________ contain slender processes of osteocytes.

a. osteoblasts
b. canaliculi
c. osteoclasts
d. glycoproteins

213. Osteoprogenitor cells and osteoblasts are found in the outer layer of bone tissue called the __________.

a. periosteum
b. lacuna
c. canaliculi
d. perichondrium

214. How many osteocytes can be found in each lucuna?

a. 1
b. 3
c. 4
d. 6

215. Which of the following is made of collagen fibers that binds the periosteum to the bone?

a. osteocyte
b. red bone marrow
c. Sharpey's fibers
d. lacuna

216. Which of the following has a function of bone resorption?

a. osteoblast
b. osteocyte
c. osteoclast
d. osteoprogenitor cells

217. The distal end of bone is called the __________, and the shaft of bone is referred to as the __________.

a. epiphysis, metaphysis
b. epiphysis, diaphysis
c. metaphysis, diaphysis
d. diaphysis, metaphysis

218. _________ joins the diaphysis to the epiphysis.

a. articular cartilage
b. yellow marrow
c. periosteum
d. metaphysis

219. Yellow bone marrow contains fat cells; it's found in the diaphysis of long bones such as the femur.

a. true
b. false

220. Which is false pertaining to primary bone tissue?

a. It has a reduced mineral content.
b. It has a greater proportion of osteocytes than secondary bone tissue
c. It is mostly replace by secondary bone tissue.
d. It is arranged is a regular arrangement of collagen fibers.

221. Immature and woven bone refer to which type of bone?
a. lamellar bone
b. mature bone
c. secondary bone
d. primary bone

222. The growth of short bones and bones of the skull are created through:
a. intramembranous ossification
b. endochondral ossification

223. The growth in the long bones is due to:
a. intramembranous ossification
b. endochondral ossification

224. The most common type of ossification is
a. endochondral
b. intramembranous

225. All of the following are formed from intramembranous ossification except:
a. mandible
b. occipital bone
c. temporal bone
d. femur

226. The growth in the width of bone is referred to as _________, and the growth in the length of bone is called _________.
a. interstitial growth, appositional growth
b. appositional growth, interstitial growth

227. Which is a function of both the endosteum and periosteum?
a. provide osteoblasts for repair
b. provide nutrition to the bone

c. provide osteoblasts for growth of bone
d. all of the above

228. The small spaces between the concentric lamellae are referred to as
a. lacunae
b. canaliculi
c. central canals
d. perforating canals

229. Haversian canals are parallel to the long axis of bone and Volkmann's canals are perpendicular to the long axis of bone.
a. true
b. false

230. Approximately 50% of bone is composed of __________.
a. water
b. protein fibers
c. mineral salts

231. Hydroxyapatite is a crystalized form of __________, which is a _________.
a. tricalcium carbonate, mineral salt
b. collagen, protein
c. fluoride, mineral salt
d. sulfate, calcification

232. Which of the following is true about collagen?
a. Collagen provides tensile strength.
b. Without collagen bone would be brittle and break easily.
c. Hardness of bone is made possible by crystallized salts & collagen.
d. All of the above

233. Which is true of compact bone?
a. located in the diaphysis of long bones
b. concentric ring structure
c. It contains Volkmann's and Haversian canals.
d. all of the above

234. All of the following are part of the osteon (Haversian system) except:
   a. canaliculi
   b. lacunae
   c. central (Haversian canal)
   d. trabeculae

235. Which types of bone contains trabeculae?
   a. spongy bone tissue
   b. dense bone tissue
   c. compact bone tissue
   d. all of the above

236. The production of bone from hyaline cartilage is called __________ ossification.
   a. intramembranous
   b. endochondral

237. The direct mineralization of matrix is a process of __________ ossification.
   a. intramembranous
   b. endochondral

238. The thickening of long bone is caused by intramembranous ossification.
   a. true
   b. false

239. Hemopoiesis is a function of bone. This is the process of blood cell production.
   a. true
   b. false

240. Capillaries of the periosteum grow into calcified cartilage that is dissolving. This __________ consists of capillaries, osteoblasts, and osteoclasts.
   a. osteocyte
   b. Haversian canal
   c. periosteal bud

d. interstitial lamellae

241. The length of bone is made possible by the epiphyseal plate.
a. true
b. false

242. Primary ossification center is responsible for the growth in the length of bone.
a. true
b. false

243. Chondrocytes are arranged in columns; they do not show hypertrophy. This is referring to the __________.
a. zone of resting cartilage
b. zone of proliferating cartilage
c. hypertrophic cartilage zone
d. zone of calcified cartilage

244. The secondary ossification center can be found at the
a. diaphysis
b. metaphysis
c. epiphysis
d. all of the above

245. When the epiphyseal plate stops growing, the length of bone _________.
a. stops growing
b. increases
c. decreases

246. Which of the following will cause a decrease in collagen synthesis by osteoblasts?
a. vitamin C deficiency
b. excessive amount of vitamin A
c. excessive amount of niacin
d. none of the above

247. Which of the following is responsible for normal bone growth?

a. human growth hormone
b. tetraiodthyronine
c. triiodothyronine
d. all of the above

248. Parathyroid hormone _________ bone resorption, and calcitonin _________ bone resorption.
a. decreases, increases
b. increases, decreases

249. Osteoclasts are increased by ___________, and osteoclasts activity is decreased by __________.
a. calcitonin, parathyroid hormone
b. parathyroid hormone, calcitonin
c. calcitonin, calcitonin
d. parathyroid hormone, parathyroid hormone

250. 99% of the calcium in the body is located in ________.
a. blood
b. skin
c. bone
d. spinal cord

251. When there is too little calcium concentration in the blood, it is taken from the bone.
a. true
b. false

252. Which is a function of bone?
a. mineral homeostasis
b. energy storage
c. hemopoiesis
d. all of the above

253. Which of the following increases the activity of osteoblasts to build bone?
a. sex hormones
b. estrogen

c. testosterone
d. all of the above

254. The first stage of fracture repair occurs approximately 7 hours after injury is referred to as
a. bony callus formation
b. remodeling
c. fibrocartilaginous callus formation
d. fracture hematoma

255. The last stage of fracture repair is ___________.
a. fibrocartilaginous callus formation
b. bony callus formation
c. remodeling
d. fracture hematoma

256. Which is the correct order of fracture repair?
a. remodeling, fracture hematoma, bony callus formation, fibrocartilaginous callus formation
b. fracture hematoma, fibrocartilaginous callus formation, bony callus formation, remodeling
c. fracture hematoma, bony callus formation, fibrocartilaginous callus formation, remodeling
d. none of the above

257. Osteoprogenitor cells develop into chondrocytes in _________ of fracture repair, which occurs approximately for 21 days.
a. fibrocartilaginous callus formation
b. bony callus formation
c. fracture hematoma
d. remodeling

258. New bone is created by ________ and old bone is destroyed by ________.
a. osteoblasts, osteoclasts
b. osteoclasts, osteoblasts
c. osteoclasts, osteocytes
d. osteoclasts, osteoprogenitor cells

259. The skeletal system is primarily developed from
   a. ectoderm
   b. endoderm
   c. mesoderm
   d. all of the above

Matching:

260. diarthrosis	a. slightly moveable joint
261. synarthrosis	b. freely moveable joint
262. amphiarthrosis	c. immovable joint
263. synovial joint	d. no joint cavity (structural classification only)
264. fibrous joint	e. has joint cavity (structural classification only)

265. All of the following are types of synarthroses except:
   a. synchondrosis
   b. gomphosis
   c. syndesmosis
   d. synostosis

266. _________ has a synovial joint with articular cartilage.
   a. synarthrosis
   b. diathrosis
   c. amphiarthrosis
   d. syndesmosis

267. All of the following are located in a diathrosis except:
   a. articular cartilage
   b. synovial joint
   c. fibrous capsule
   d. cartilaginous joint

268. The articular capsule is composed of the outer __________ and inner _________.
   a. fibrous capsule, synovial membrane
   b. synovial membrane, fibrous capsule
   c. articular cartilage, synovial fluid
   d. synovial fluid, articular cartilage

269. The synovial membrane is composed of

a. areolar connective tissue
b. adipose tissue
c. elastic fibers
d. all of the above

270. Type A cells line the synovial membrane and are similar to __________ . Type B cells of the synovial membrane are similar to __________.

a. phagocytes, fibroblasts
b. fibroblasts, phagocytes

Nerve Tissue

271. The cell body is referred to as the ________.

a. dendrite
b. axon
c. perikaryon
d. synapse

272. Which of the following is composed of the neuron?

a. cell body
b. axon
c. dendrites
d. all of above

273. Where does the axon connect to the cell body of a neuron?

a. Nissl body
b. axon hillock
c. dendrite
d. axon collateral

274. Which of the following is part of the cytoplasm of the dendrite that is responsible for protein synthesis?

a. Nissl body
b. axon hillock
c. axon
d. white matter

275. Nissl bodies are made of an array of __________ and free ribosomes.
   a. rough endoplasmic reticulum
   b. dendrites
   c. mitochondria
   d. centrosomes

276. Which is an unmyelinated branched process that is found around the cell body of a neuron?
   a. axon
   b. Schwann cell
   c. myelin sheath
   d. dendrite

277. Which of the following forms the cytoskeleton of a nerve cell?
   a. chromatophilic substance
   b. dendrite
   c. neurofibril
   d. axon hillock

278. ________ is described as an axon or dendrite.
   a. myelin sheath
   b. neurofibril
   c. axon hillock
   d. nerve fiber

279. All of the following consists of gray matter except:
   a. myelinated processes
   b. dendrites
   c. unmylinated axons
   d. axon terminals

280. Which of the following is found around axons in the PNS?
   a. neurolemma
   b. dendrites
   c. axon hillock
   d. axon terminals

281. Nerve tissue develops from

a. mesoderm
b. endoderm
c. ectoderm

282. End bulbs of a neuron interact with other neurons to form _________.
a. axon terminals
b. terminal arborizations
c. synapses
d. neurofibrils

283. Which of the following types of neurons have only one process and is sensory only?
a. pseudounipolar neuron
b. bipolar neuron
c. multipolar neuron
d. all of the above

284. Which of the following are the most common type of neurons?
a. pseudounipolar
b. multipolar
c. bipolar

285. ________ gives rise to the entire central nervous system.
a. neural tube
b. neural crest
c. dendrite
d. axon

286. Which part of the neuron has a function of receiving information from other neurons and sensory epithelial cells?
a. axon
b. myelin
c. end bulbs
d. dendrite

287. Most of the peripheral nervous system is derived from the _________.
a. axon
b. dendrite

c. neural crest
d. neural tube

288. All of the following are located in the central nervous system except:
a. oligodendroctye
b. ependymal cell
c. Schwann cell
d. astrocyte

289. Which of the following consists of the central nervous system?
a. spinal cord
b. cerebrum
c. cerebellum
d. all of the above

290. _________ create myelin in the peripheral nervous system around axons.
a. oligodendrocytes
b. Schwann cells
c. astrocytes
d. microglia

291. The spaces between axons that are not myelinated are called:
a. axon collaterals
b. nodes of Ravier
c. Schwann cells
d. axon hillocks

292. _________ creates myelin in the central nervous system; it provides electric insulation.
a. astrocyte
b. microglia
c. Schwann cell
d. oligodendrocyte

293. ________ are known as phagocytic neuroglia that develop from monocytes.
a. astrocytes

b. microglia
c. oligodendroctyes
d. myelin sheath

294. Which of the following is a principle type of cell that supports and protects the neurons?
a. glia cells
b. neuroglia
c. dendrites
d. both a and b

295. Which of the following transmits impulses to other neurons?
a. dendrite
b. axon
c. microglia
d. Nissl bodies

296. Which is not true of the astrocyte?
a. helps in the formation of the blood-brain barrier
b. It is found in the gray matter of the central nervous system.
c. It binds neurons to the pia mater.
d. It produces myelin sheath in the peripheral nervous system.

297. __ ____ are composed of epithelial cells that line the ventricles of the brain.
a. Schwann cells
b. ependymal cells
c. microglia
d. astrocytes

298. All of the following are types of neuroglia?
a. microglia
b. satellite cells
c. ependymal cells
d. all of the above

299. Which type of glial cell (neuroglia) encircles neuronal cell bodies in the peripheral nervous system?

a. satellite cells
b. Schwann cells
c. Ependymal cells
d. dendtrites

300. Which type of glial cell (neuroglia) has a function as a macrophage that destroys bacteria in the central nervous system?
a. Schwann cells
b. satellite cells
c. ependymal cells
d. microglia

301. ________ is a type of meninges that is made of dense, irregular connective tissue that is closest to the skull.
a. dura mater
b. pia mater
c. arachnoid
d. subarachnoid space

302. The ________ is the inner layer of the meninges; it is separated from the spinal cord and nerve tissue by neuroglial processes.
a. arachnoid
b. dura mater
c. pia mater
d. subarachnoid space

303. The outer layer of the meninges is called the _________.
a. pia mater
b. dura mater
c. arachnoid
d. subarachnoid space

304. The brain is enclosed by meninges. However, the spinal cord is only encircled by the subarchnoid space.
a. true
b. false
The brain and spinal cord are enclosed by the meninges. The correct answer is B.

305. Which of the following is wrapped around an axon which serves as insulation and increases the speed of a nerve impulse?

a. dendrite
b. astrocyte
c. myelin sheath
d. microglia

306. Which of the following is a cell inclusion that is located in the nerve cell?

a. Nissl body
b. golgi complex
c. mitochondria
d. lipofuscin

Lipofuscin is a pigment, which comes from the undigested material of a lysosome. Cell inclusions are not bounded by membranes. The correct answer is D.

307. Efferent neurons transmit impulses from the spinal cord and brain to the muscles. Afferent neurons transmit sensory impulses from outside the CNS to the spinal cord and brain.

a. true
b. false

308. Efferent neurons are _________, and afferent neurons are _________.

a. sensory, motor
b. motor, sensory

309. Meninges are generally covered by which type of epithelia?

a. simple columnar
b. simple squamous
c. transitional
d. stratified columnar

310. Simple squamous epithelium that covers the dura mater is developed from _________.

a. ectoderm
b. endoderm

c. mesenchyme

311. All of the following are the meninges except:
a. dura mater
b. subdural space
c. pia mater
d. arachnoid

312. Gray matter consists of all of the following except:
a. neuronal cell bodies
b. dendrites
c. unmyelinated parts of axons and glial cells
d. myelinated axons

313. White matter generally consists of myelinated cells while gray matter is absent of myelination.
a. true
b. false

314. The majority of synapses are __________, which transmit impulses by neurotransmitters.
a. electric
b. chemical
c. unmyelinated
d. none of the above

315. The three functions of the nervous system are integrative, _________, and _________.
a. motor, sensory
b. motor, peripheral
c. sensory, peripheral
d. none of the above

316. Which type of cell is is made of reticular fibers that are produced by Schwann cells?
a. perineurium
b. epineurium
c. endoneurium

d. satellite cells

317. Which type surrounds the entire nerve?
a. perineurium
b. epineurium
c. endoneurium
d. spinal cord

318. Each bundle of nerve fibers are directly surrounded by the __________.
a. endoneurium
b. epineurium
c. perineurium
d. axon

319. Each nerve fiber is surrounded directly by the ___________.
a. axon
b. perineurium
c. epineurium
d. endoneurium

320. Bundle of nerve fibers are called
a. axons
b. fascicles
c. epineurium
d. perineurium

321. Most nerves are ________ nerves.
a. sensory
b. motor
c. mixed
d. efferent

322. The choroid plexus is composed of capillaries and _________.
a. dura mater
b. pia mater
c. arachnoid
d. subdural space

323. All of the following are made of the choroid plexus except:
   a. simple cuboidal epithelium
   b. loose connective tissue of the pia mater
   c. low columnar epithelium
   d. loose connective tissue of the dura mater

324. Pia mater consists of
   a. reticular fibers
   b. collagen fibers
   c. blood vessels
   d. all of the above

325. Which of the following is not part of the peripheral nervous system?
   a. spinal cord
   b. ganglia
   c. nerve endings
   d. nerves

Muscle Tissue & Tissue of the Circulatory System

326. Muscle tissue is primarily derived from:
   a. ectoderm
   b. mesoderm
   c. endoderm
   d. neural groove

327. Which type of muscle is involuntary and consists of fusiform fibers?
   a. skeletal
   b. cardiac
   c. smooth
   d. all of the above

328. Intercalated disks are observed in ________ muscle.
   a. cardiac
   b. smooth
   c. skeletal
   d. none of the above

329. Which of the following is a voluntary type of muscle tissue?

a. skeletal
b. smooth
c. cardiac
d. all of the above

330. ________ muscle does not have cross-striations.

a. cardiac
b. skeletal
c. smooth
d. none of the above

331. Troponin consists of which of the following subunits?

a. TnT
b. TnT
c. TnC
d. all of the above

332. Troponin has the subunit ________, which binds to calcium ions.

a. TnT
b. TnC
c. TnI
d. all of the above

333. TnI prevents the actin-myosin interaction.

a. true
b. false

334. Which of the following is the primary protein of intermediate filaments in smooth muscle?

a. desmin
b. glycogen
c. tropomyosin
d. troponin

335. In multiple innervation, a motor unit consists of one nerve fiber and the muscles it innervates.

a. true

b. false

336. Which of the following shortens during a muscle contraction?
a. myosin
b. actin
c. sacromere
d. only thick filament

337. _______ and tropomyosin stop myosin cross bridges from binding with actin.
a. titin
b. troponin
c. intercalated discs
d. calmodulin

338. Cross bridges refer to the ________
a. actin tail
b. actin head
c. myosin tail
d. myosin head

339. Which of the following are slow twitch fibers that do not fatigue easily?
a. type II A fibers
b. type I fibers
c. type II b fibers
d. fast twitch fibers

340. _______ is mobilized during a muscle contraction for energy.
a. glycogen
b. myoglobin
c. hemoglobin
d. all of the above

341. Which of the following is a membrane enclosed tubule that stores calcium for contraction?
a. sarcolemma
b. cytoplasm

c. sarcoplasmic reticulum
d. calmodulin

342. Which type of muscle fiber is least resistant to fatigue and is located primarily in the muscles of the arms?
a. type I fibers
b. type II A fibers
c. type II B fibers
d. slow twitch fibers

343. Troponin and tropomyosin are regulatory proteins blocking the myosin binding sites on ________.
a. titin
b. myosin
c. actin
d. elastic filament

344. Troponin and Tropomyosin block the myosin binding sites on action during ________.
a. muscle contraction
b. muscle relaxation

345. All of the following are thin filaments except:
a. myosin
b. actin
c. troponin
d. tropomyosin

346. Which of the following is a regulatory protein in smooth muscle?
a. troponin
b. calmodulin
c. tropomyosin
d. all of the above

347. Which type of muscle has the fastest speed of contraction?
a. smooth muscle
b. skeletal muscle
c. cardiac muscle

348. Z disc to Z disc is approximately one
   a. sacromere
   b. I band
   c. sarcoplasmic reticulum
   d. sarcoplasm

349. The contractile parts of skeletal muscles are called:
   a. sarcolemma
   b. sarcoplasma
   c. motor units
   d. myofibrils

350. Myofibrils consist of _________ filaments.
   a. elastic
   b. thin
   c. thick
   d. all of the above

351. Each muscle bundle is directly surrounded by the ________.
   a. perimysium
   b. endomysium
   c. epimysium
   d. none of the above

352. Each muscle fiber is surrounded by the ________, which is composed of reticular fibers and basal lamina.
   a. epimysium
   b. endomysium
   c. perimysium

353. The _ ___ encircles the entire muscle; it is made of dense connective tissue.
   a. endomysium
   b. perimysium
   c. epimysium

354. Which of the following is false pertaining to smooth muscle?
   a. it is non-striated

b. smooth muscle is smallest at the midpoint and largest at the ends
c. they are fusiform
d. they are encircled by basal lamina and reticular fibers

355. Smooth muscle is innervated by
a. parasympathetic nervous system
b. sympathetic nervous system
c. both a and b

356. Dense bodies in smooth muscle are most similar to _______ in striated muscle.
a. Z discs
b. M lines
c. I bands
d. H zones

357. ________ is a regulatory protein that binds calcium in the cytosol in non-striated muscle; _________ is a regulatory protein that binds calcium in the cytosol in striated muscle.
a. calmodulin, troponin
b. troponin, calmodulin
c. troponin, tropomyosin
d. tropmyosin, troponin

358. All of the following are true regarding visceral (single-unit) smooth muscle tissue except:
a. It forms a portion of the walls of small arteries and veins.
b. It is found in hollow viscera.
c. It contracts as a single unit.
d. It is the least common type of smooth muscle.

359. All of the following are locations for visceral smooth muscle tissue except:
a. urinary bladder
b. uterus
c. stomach
d. radial and circular muscles of the iris of the eye

360. Which of the following has the greatest capacity for regeneration?
a. smooth muscle
b. skeletal muscle
c. cardiac muscle
d. all of the above

361. Which of the following has the no capacity for regeneration?
a. smooth muscle
b. skeletal muscle
c. cardiac muscle
d. all of the above

362. ________ has no sacromeres or transverse tubules.
a. smooth muscle
b. skeletal muscle
c. cardiac muscle
d. all of the above have sacromeres only

363. Which of the following has no gap junctions with a very large fiber diameter?
a. cardiac muscle
b. smooth muscle
c. skeletal muscle
d. all of the above

364. Where are multiunit smooth muscles found in the body?
a. arrector pili muscles
b. large blood vessels
c. muscles of the iris
d. all of the above

365. Multiunit smooth muscles contract
a. independently
b. together at the same time

366. Which of the following can smooth muscle synthesize?
a. collagen
b. proteoglycan

c. elastin
d. all of the above

367. The cell membrane of muscles tissue is called the
a. sarcoplasm
b. sarcolemma
c. sarcomere
d. sarcoplasmic reticulum

368. The cytoplasm of muscle tissue is called
a. sarcolemma
b. sarcoplasm
c. sarcomere
d. plasmalemma

369. Which of the following is a layer of blood vessels?
a. tunica media
b. tunica intima
c. tunica adventitia
d. all of the above

370. ________ separates the tunica media from the tunica adventitia in large arteries.
a. tunica intima
b. internal elastic lamina
c. external elastic lamina
d. endothelium

371. The most outer layer of blood vessels is referred to as the
a. tunica adventitia
b. tunica intima
c. tunica media
d. external elastic lamina

372. Which is the inner layer of blood vessels?
a. tunica media
b. tunica intima
c. tunica adventitia

d. internal elastic lamina

373. The tunica media is made of _________.

a. concentric layers of smooth muscle cells
b. endothelial cells
c. subendothelial layer
d. all of the above

374. Which of the following separates the tunica intima from the tunica media?

a. tuncia adventitia
b. subendothelial layer
c. internal elastic lamina
d. external elastic lamina

375. The collagen in tunica adventitia is primarily of which type?

a. Type I
b. Type II
c. Type III
d. Type IV

376. The thickest layer in veins is usually the

a. tunica adventitia
b. tunica media
c. tunica intima

377. The tunica media is replaced by ________ in the capillaries of the body.

a. fenestrae
b. pericytes
c. endothelial cells
d. subendothelial layer

378. Which of the following contains elastic fibers and smooth fiber muscle cells in this thickest layer of the tunics pertaining to arteries?

a. tunica interna
b. tunica media
c. tunica adventitia

d. all of the above

379. Capillaries are composed of which of the following layers?
a. layer of endothelial cells
b. tunica adventitia
c. tunica media
d. type I collagen fibers

380. Which is a type of capillary?
a. fenestrated
b. continuous
c. sinusoidal
d. all of the above

381. In arteries, the internal elastic lamina that distinguishes the tunica intima from the tunica lamina has gaps called fenestrae.
a. true
b. false

382. The endothelium is composed of simple squamous epithelium.
a. true
b. false

383. Capillaries consist of an endothelial layer and _________.
a. tunica media
b. tunica externa
c. basement membrane
d. external elastic lamina

384. Sinusoidal capillaries are found primarily in the _________.
a. liver
b. bone marrow
c. spleen
d. none of the above

385. Sinusoidal capillaries are located in the ________.
a. spleen
b. liver

c. bone marrow
d. all of the above

386. Many capillaries unite to form _________, which are small veins.
a. arterioles
b. venules
c. veins
d. pulmonary vessels

387. The walls of arteries are generally thinner compared to veins.
a. true
b. false

388. Which of the following statements is false?
a. The lumen of a vein is larger than the lumen of the artery.
b. The thickest portion of vein is tunica adventitia.
c. The tunics in veins are thinner than the tunics in arteries.
d. Veins only have only two layers: tunica adventitia and tunica media

389. Arteries bring blood directly into capillaries.
a. true
b. false

390. Which layer of the heart is the thickest and is responsible for heart pumping?
a. epicardium
b. myocardium
c. endocardium
d. serous covering of the heart

391. Which serves as the site of insertion and origin for cardiac muscles?
a. fibrous skeleton
b. myocardium
c. collagen
d. gap junctions

392. The visceral layer of the serous pericardium is referred to as the:
a. tunics

b. endocardium
c. myocardium
d. epicardium

393. The epicardium is covered by which type of epithelium?
a. transitional
b. simple squamous
c. simple cuboidal
d. columnar

394. Purkinje cells can be located in the subendocardial layer of the heart.
a. true
b. false

395. Which is not a component of the fibrous skeleton of the heart?
a. septum membranaceum
b. annuli fibrosi
c. trigona fibrosa
d. all of the above

396. The endocardium is most similar to the
a. tunica adventitia
b. tunica media
c. tunica intima
d. fibrous skeleton

Blood cells and Hematopoiesis

397. The primary function of neutrophils is which of the following?
a. defense against viruses
b. phagocytosis of bacteria
c. blood clotting
d. histamine production

398. All of the following are granular leukocytes except:
a. eosinophils
b. basophils
c. neutrophils

d. lymphoctyes

399. Which plasma protein plays an important role in blood clotting?
a. fibrinogen
b. gamma globulin
c. alpha globulin
d. albumin

400. The most abundant plasma protein is:
a. fibrinogen
b. gamma globulin
c. alpha globulin
d. albumin

401. Whole blood is made of blood plasma and formed elements. Approximately 99% of all formed elements are __________.
a. red blood cells
b. neutrophils
c. lymphoctyes
d. basophils

402. The process of _________ formation is called erythropoiesis.
a. basophile
b. red blood cell
c. T cell
d. B cell

403. All of the following are agranuloctyes except:
a. T cells
b. B cells
c. basophils
d. lymphocytes

404. __________ serves specifically as a defense against parasitic infection.
a. erythrocytes
b. eosinophils
c. T lymphocytes

d. platelets

405. All of the following are formed elements of the blood except:
a. thrombocytes
b. lymphocytes
c. fibrinogen
d. granuloctye

406. Which of the following is a formed element of blood?
a. erythrocytes
b. leukocytes
c. platelets
d. all of the above

407. The young erythrocyte is called the
a. reticulocyte
b. monocyte
c. lymphocyte
d. granulocyte

408. Which is the correct order of red blood cell production (from earliest to latest)?
a. rubriblast, rubricyte, prorubricyte, metarubricyte
b. rubriblast, prorubrictye, rubricyte, metarubricyte
c. metarubricyte, rubricyte, prorubrictye, rubriblast
d. rubricyte, metarubricyte, prorubricyte, rubriblast

409. Red blood cell usually have a life span of approximately
a. 24 hours
b. 60 days
c. 120 days
d. 7 days

410. Oxygen transport is a primary function of:
a. white blood cells
b. red blood cells
c. fibrinogen
d. neutrophil

411. Which of the following forms platelets?
a. myeloblasts
b. monoblasts
c. megakaryoblasts
d. lymphoblasts

412. ________ is a pluripotent hematopoietic stem cell, which is derived from ________.
a. erythoblast, ectoderm
b. reticulocyte, endoderm
c. monocyte, ectoderm
d. hemocytoblast, mesenchyme

413. Which is a false statement pertaining to red blood cells?
a. They are biconcave.
b. Sickle-cell anemia gives rise to inflexible and delicate red blood cells.
c. Red blood cells have an average life span of 120 days.
d. Erythrocytes make up part of the blood plasma.

414. Proerythroblasts, myeloblasts, monoblasts, megakaryoblasts, and lymphoblasts are all directed derived from:
a. hemocytoblasts
b. erythrocytes
c. monocytes
d. thrombocytes

415. The red color of blood comes from which oxygen carrying pigment?
a. platelets
b. hemoglobulin
c. fibrinogen
d. T cells

416. The most abundant type of leukocyte is the __________.
a. eosinophil
b. basophil
c. lymphocyte
d. neutrophil

417. The least abundant leukocyte is the _________.
   a. lymphoctye
   b. eosinophil
   c. basophil
   d. monocyte

418. Approximately 5% of all leukocytes are
   a. lymphocytes
   b. monocytes
   c. eosinophils
   d. basophils

419. Neutrophils and monocytes function greatly in phagocytosis.
   a. true
   b. false

420. Granulocytes are considered ____________.
   a. polymorphonuclear leukocytes
   b. mononuclear leukocytes

421. All of the following polymorphonuclear leukocytes except:
   a. lymphoctyes
   b. neutrophils
   c. eosinophils
   d. basophils

422. Which is the correct order of development of a thrombocyte?
   a. megakaryocyte, metamegakaryocyte, promegakaryocyte, thrombocyte
   b. promegakaryocyte, megakaryocyte, metamegakaryocyte, thrombocyte
   c. megakaryocyte, promegakaryocyte, metamegakaryocyte, thrombocyte

423. _______ aids the platelet in maintaining its shape.
   a. open canalicular system
   b. neutrophil
   c. marginal bundle of microtubules

d. all of the above

424. The platelet has a function of
a. repairing gaps in wall of blood vessels
b. blood clotting
c. both a and b
d. parasitic defense

425. Older neutrophils are called _________; they have nuclei with many shapes.
a. bands
b. polymorphonuclear leukocytes
c. T cells
d. B cells

426. High amounts of eosinophils in the blood occur with
a. allergic reactions
b. Niacin deficiency

427. The process of blood cell formation is referred to as:
a. monocytopoiesis
b. erythropoiesis
c. megakaryocytopoiesis
d. hematopoiesis

428. Hematopoiesis occurs in the _________ after birth.
a. yolk sac
b. red bone marrow

429. Hematopoiesis occurs in the lymph nodes, thymus, and _________ during embryonic development.
a. yolk sac
b. liver
c. spleen
d. all of the above

430. The bone marrow produces cells called _________ that will move to the lymphoid organs to eventually produce B cells and T cells.

a. lymphoid multipotential cells
b. myeloid multipotential cells
c. promonocytes
d. eosinophils

431. Promonocytes directly derive from the __________ and the promyelocytes derive from ________.
a. lymphoblasts, megakaryoblasts
b. proerythroblasts, myeloblasts
c. monoblasts, myeloblasts
d. metamyelocyte, monoblasts

432. Myeloid multipotential cells and lymphoid multipotential cells originate from the ________.
a. lymphoblast
b. megakaryoblast
c. pluripotential cell
d. eosinophilic granulocyte

433. Which of the following is a stem cell in the bone marrow that can make all blood cell types?
a. lymphoid multipotential cell
b. pluripotential cell
c. myeloid multipotential cell
d. megakaryoblast

434. _________ are mature cells that do not undergo mitotic activity.
a. lymphoblasts
b. monocytes
c. megakaryocyte-forming cell
d. erythroblast

435. _______ is produced by the ________ ; this hormone will increase the rate of growth from a proerythroblast to a reticulocyte.
a. erythropoietin, kidneys
b. erythropoietin, stomach
c. hermosiderin, kidneys
d. hermosiderin, stomach

436. Promyelocytes differentiate into all of the following except:
   a. eosinophilic myelocyte
   b. neutrophilic myelocyte
   c. basophilic myelocyte
   d. prolymphocyte

437. The primary location of hematopoiesis in the body is the ________.
   a. spleen
   b. liver
   c. bone marrow
   d. lymph nodes

438. Red bone marrow is located in the
   a. medullary canal of long bones
   b. cancellous bone
   c. both a and b

Lymphoid Organs

439. All of the following are lymphoid organs except:
   a. spleen
   b. thymus
   c. lymph nodes
   d. stomach

440. T lymphocytes mature in the _________; they first come from the ________.
   a. thymus, bone marrow
   b. spleen, thymus
   c. thymus, spleen
   d. bone marrow, spleen

441. All of the following are considered peripheral lymphoid organs except:
   a. appendix
   b. tonsils
   c. lymphoid nodes
   d. thymus

442. The thymus and the ________ are central lymphoid organs.

a. appendix
b. Peyer's patches
c. bone marrow
d. spleen

443. Which of the following is peripheral lymphoid organ?

a. bone marrow
b. spleen
c. thymus
d. all of the above

444. B lymphocytes become mature cells in the bone marrow.

a. true
b. false

445. B lymphocytes are derived from the ________.

a. spleen
b. bone marrow
c. appendix
d. Peyer's patches

446. The greatest percentage of T lymphocytes is found in the ________.

a. bone marrow
b. thymus
c. spleen
d. lymph nodes

447. The greatest percentage of B lymphocytes is in which lympoid organ?

a. spleen
b. thymus
c. bone marrow
d. blood

448. The ________ is a ________ lymphoid organ that consists of a red and white pulp.

a. spleen, peripheral
b. thymus, central

c. tonsils, peripheral
d. spleen, central

449. The Billroth's cords are located in the _________ of the _________.
a. white pulp, spleen
b. red pulp, spleen
c. red pulp, thymus
d. white pulp, thymus

450. Dense connective tissue is located around the spleen, which has a marginal zone that separates the red and white pulp.
a. true
b. false

451. The white pulp of the spleen consists of ________ tissue, and the red pulp is a type of ________ tissue.
a. reticular, lymphoid
b. lymphoid, reticular

452. Which is a type of tonsil?
a. lingual
b. palatine
c. pharyngeal
d. all of the above

453. All of the following are true except:
a. The spleen is the location of T cell maturation.
b. The largest mass of lymphatic tissue is located in the spleen.
c. Phagocytosis of bacteria occurs in the spleen.
d. Blood is stored in the spleen.

454. Which is derived from the pluripotential cell?
a. B cell
b. T cell
c. both a and b

455. Lymphoid organs other than the thymus originate from the
a. endoderm

b. ectoderm
c. mesoderm

456. The cortex, medulla and Hassall's corpuscles are located in which organ?
a. blood
b. spleen
c. thymus
d. tonsils

457. The cortex of the medulla consists of:
a. macrophages
b. T lymphocytes
c. epithelial reticular cells
d. all of the above

458. Hassall's corpuscles are found in the ________ of the ________.
a. red pulp, spleen
b. white pulp, spleen
c. cortex, thymus
d. cortex, thymus

459. The cortex and the medulla of the ______ consists of reticular epithelial cells. The ________ does not contain Hassall's corpuscles.
a. thymus, cortex
b. thymus, medulla
c. spleen, cortex
d. spleen, red pulp

460. All of the following are components of the spleen except:
a. red pulp
b. white pulp
c. marginal zone sinuses
d. medulla

461. Approximately 12 % of lymphocytes are _________ , which have a primary function of destroying virus-infected cells and cancer cells.
a. T lymphocytes

b. B lymphocytes
c. natural killer lymphocytes
d. neutrophils

462. Which leukocyte differentiates into a plasma cell?
a. T lymphocyte
b. monocyte
c. B lymphocyte
d. eosinophil

463. Antigens stimulate B and T cells to make immunoblasts.
a. true
b. false

Matching:

464. Outer cortex	a. separates medullary cords
465. Medullary lymphoid sinuses	b. contains reticular fibers, cortical sinus, and lymphoid nodules
466. Medulla	c. inner area of the lymph node
467. Spleen	d. contains Hassall's corpuscles
468. Thymus	e. biggest mass of lymphatic tissue

469. Splenic cords are found in the red pulp; they contain
a. plasma cells
b. granulocytes
c. macrophages
d. all of the above

470. Which of the following is a function of the spleen?
a. eradication of red blood cells
b. formation of lymphoctyes
c. store blood
d. all of the above

471. The lingual tonsils are covered by ________ epithelium.
a. simple squamous
b. stratified squamous
c. transitional

d. none of the above

472. All of the following are true pertaining to lymph nodes except:
   a. They can be rounded or kidney shaped organs.
   b. Lymph nodes have a medulla and cortex.
   c. Lymph nodes are considered central lymphoid organs.
   d. Medullary lymphoid sinuses contain lymph.

Digestive System

473. Water absorption takes place in the large intestine.
   a. true
   b. false

474. Which is the outermost layer of most portions of the gastrointestinal tract?
   a. mucosa
   b. submucosa
   c. serosa
   d. muscularis

475. The most inner layer of the gastrointestinal tract is the _________.
   a. serosa
   b. muscularis
   c. submucosa
   d. mucosa

476. The serosa is composed of simple squamous epithelium.
   a. true
   b. false

477. The muscularis is a layer of the digestive tract that contains only smooth muscle.
   a. true
   b. false

Muscularis also contains skeletal muscle. B is the correct answer.

478. Which is the outer layer of the mucosa?

a. muscularis
b. muscularis mucosae
c. serosa
d. lamina propria

479. The mesothelium is directly around the _________.
a. muscularis
b. serosa
c. lamina propria
d. muscularis mucosae

480. The cardia, fundus and body are all regions of the ________.
a. large intestine
b. esophagus
c. stomach
d. small intestine

481. All of the following are layers of the mucosa except:
a. lamina propria
b. epithelium layer in direct connection with contents of GI tract
c. muscularis mucosae
d. serosa

482. Which of the following is not a region of the small intestine?
a. jejunum
b. duodenum
c. ileum
d. pylorus

483. Which is the most superficial layer of the GI tract?
a. serosa
b. mucosa
c. muscularis
d. submucosa

484. The _________ of the tongue are covered with projections of lamina propria and epithelium.
a. papillae

b. stomach
c. small intestine
d. large intestine

485. The pharnyx consists of which type of epithelium?
a. pseudostratified columnar
b. squamous
c. transitional
d. both a and b

486. Pepsinogen is a precursor of pepsin; it is secreted by _________ cells, which are found in the _________.
a. parietal, stomach
b. chief, stomach
c. G, small intestine
d. mucous, small intestine

487. Which is a type of cell found in the gastric glands?
a. parietal cells
b. mucous cells
c. G cells
d. chief cells
e. all of the above

488. Which of the following creates peristalsis in the stomach?
a. mucosa
b. muscularis

489. _________ cells secrete hydrochoric acid. In this way, most bacteria in food is destroyed.
a. chief
b. zymogenic
c. mucous
d. parietal

490. Parietal cells secrete __________ so vitamin B12 can be absorbed.
a. intrinsic factor
b. hydrochloric acid

c. pepsin
d. pepsinogen

491. Gastrin is secreted by the ________ cells of the stomach.
a. mucous
b. G
c. oxyntic
d. zymogenic

492. The crypts of Lieberkuhn are __________ glands found in the ________.
a. small intestinal, mucosa
b. pancreatic, mucosa
c. stomach, submucosa
d. stomach, muscularis

493. Which of the following increases the surface area of the intestines?
a. microvilli
b. villi
c. plicae
d. all of the above

494. Goblet cells are located in the small intestine.
a. true
b. false

495. Which cell located in the small intestine secretes lysosyme, which helps in destroying bacteria?
a. Paneth cells
b. Goblet cells
c. M cells
d. Zymogenic cells

Matching:

496. pancreas	a. contains Kupffer's cells
497. liver	b. contains islets of Langerhans
498. gallbladder	c. stores bile
499. small intestine	d. location of taeniae coli

500. large intestine e. major place of digestion

501. The islets of Langerhans make up the _________ part of the pancreas; they secrete ________.

a. exocrine, insulin
b. exocrine, gastrin
c. endocrine, gastrin
d. endocrine, insulin

502. The exocrine part of the pancreas is made of __________.

a. acini
b. islets of Langerhans
c. Glisson's capsule
d. parietal cells

503. The liver has an outside covering composed of a structure called:

a. islets of Langerhans
b. Glisson's capsule
c. ampulla of Vater
d. submucosa

504. Which of the following is a type of papilla?

a. fungiform
b. circumvallate
c. filiform
d. all of the above

505. The serosa is superficial to the ________ layer of the GI tract.

a. mucosa
b. submucosa
c. muscularis
d. all of the above

506. All of the following are accessory structures of the GI tract except:

a. teeth
b. pancreas
c. liver
d. pharynx

507. All of the following are accessory structures of the GI tract that never come in contact with food except:

a. pharynx
b. pancreas
c. gallbladder
d. salivary glands

508. The hardest part of the body is:

a. bone
b. dentin
c. enamel
d. gingiva

509. Which of the following contains the most calcium salts?

a. bone
b. enamel
c. dentin
d. gingiva

510. The matrix of dentin is secreted by _________, and the matrix of enamel is secreted by ________.

a. odontoblasts, ameloblasts
b. ameloblasts, odontoblasts
c. osteoblasts, odontoblasts
d. ameloblasts, osteoblasts

511. The periodental ligament is composed of dense fibrous connective tissue.

a. true
b. false

512. Most structures of the teeth are derived from _________. However, enamel is derived from _________.

a. ectoderm, endoderm
b. endoderm, ectoderm
c. mesoderm, ectoderm
d. endoderm, mesoderm

Urinary System

513. The urinary bladder consists of ________ epithelium.
a. simple columar
b. transitional
c. simple squamous
d. stratified squamous

514. Bowman's capsule surrounds which of the following structures?
a. Loop of Henle
b. collecting duct
c. thick ascending limb
d. glomerulus

515. The descending and ascending limbs compose the __________.
a. Loop of Henle
b. glomerulus
c. Bowman's capsule
d. renal pelvis

516. The loop of Henle is shaped like the letter _________.
a. N
b. U
c. A
d. C

517. The functional unit of the kidney is referred to as the ________.
a. cortex
b. glomerulus
c. nephron
d. medulla

518. Which of the following layers is found around the kidneys?
a. renal capsule
b. renal fascia
c. adipose capsule
d. all of the above

519. Blood plasma is filtered by the Bowman's capsule.

a. true
b. false

520. Bowman's capsule has a parietal layer that consists of _________ epithelium.

a. simple squamous
b. simple columnar
c. stratified columnar
d. stratified squamous

521. Which of the following separates the parietal and visceral layers of the glomerular capsule?

a. Bowman's space
b. proximal convoluted tubule
c. podocyte
d. brush border

522. The distal convoluted tubule is considered the ________ part of the nephron; it is composed of __________ epithelium.

a. first, transitional
b. last, transitional
c. first, simple squamous
d. last, simple cuboidal

523. Which type of cell forms the visceral layer of the glomerular capsule?

a. intercalated cells
b. podocytes
c. principle cells
d. nephron

524. The descending limb of the loop of Henle is made of ________epithelium.

a. simple cuboidal
b. simple squamous
c. transitional
d. stratified cuboidal

525. The macula densa and the juxtaglomerular cells comprise the ________.

a. glomerulus
b. Bowman's capsule
c. podocytes
d. juxtaglomerular apparatus

526. The afferent arteriole having juxtaglomerular cells is right next to the __________ of the distal convoluted tubules.

a. papillary duct
b. cortex
c. macula densa
d. glomerulus

527. Which of the following is part of the juxtaglomerular apparatus?

a. macula densa
b. extraglomerular mesangial cells
c. JG cells
d. all of the above

528. The glomerulus and Bowman's capsule are considered the _________.

a. renal tubule
b. renal corpuscle
c. renal papilla
d. collecting duct

Answers:

1. a
2. d
3. b
4. a
5. c
6. a
7. d
8. a
9. b
10. d
11. a
12. d
13. d
14. c
15. d
16. b
17. a
18. b
19. a
20. b
21. b
22. c
23. c
24. d
25. d
26. d
27. a
28. c
29. b
30. a
31. c
32. a
33. a
34. b
35. a
36. d
37. c
38. a
39. a
40. c
41. c
42. b
43. b
44. a
45. b
46. d
47. e
48. b
49. a
50. d
51. b
52. a
53. c
54. d
55. b
56. d
57. c
58. a
59. d
60. c
61. a
62. b
63. d
64. e
65. a
66. d
67. a
68. b
69. a
70. c
71. a
72. d
73. b
74. c
75. a
76. c
77. d
78. a
79. b
80. a
81. d
82. a
83. a
84. c
85. a
86. c
87. a
88. b
89. e
90. d
91. a
92. a
93. c
94. a
95. b
96. b
97. a
98. e
99. a
100. a
101. d
102. a
103. a
104. d
105. d
106. a
107. b
108. d
109. a
110. b
111. c
112. a
113. b
114. e
115. d
116. d
117. a
118. b
119. b
120. c
121. d
122. d
123. a
124. c
125. d
126. d
127. a
128. b
129. d
130. d
131. a
132. b
133. c
134. d
135. c
136. a
137. b
138. d
139. a
140. b
141. b
142. a
143. d
144. c
145. d
146. c
147. a
148. c
149. b
150. a
151. c
152. b
153. d
154. a
155. b
156. b
157. e
158. a
159. a
160. c
161. d
162. c
163. c
164. d
165. d
166. a
167. a
168. b
169. c
170. d
171. a
172. a
173. b
174. d
175. a
176. b
177. b
178. b
179. d
180. a
181. c
182. a
183. d
184. a
185. a
186. c
187. a
188. b
189. b
190. a
191. b
192. d
193. c
194. b
195. a
196. d
197. d
198. c
199. b
200. a
201. b
202. c
203. d
204. a
205. c
206. a
207. b
208. c
209. d
210. d
211. a
212. b
213. a
214. a
215. c
216. c
217. b
218. d
219. a
220. d
221. d
222. a

223. b
224. a
225. d
226. b
227. d
228. a
229. a
230. c
231. a
232. d
233. d
234. d
235. a
236. b
237. a
238. a
239. a
240. c
241. a
242. a
243. b
244. c
245. a
246. a
247. d
248. b
249. b
250. c
251. a
252. d
253. d
254. d
255. c
256. b
257. a
258. a
259. c
260. b
261. c
262. a
263. e
264. d
265. c
266. b
267. d
268. a
269. d
270. a
271. c
272. d
273. b
274. a
275. a
276. d
277. c
278. d
279. a
280. a
281. c
282. c
283. a
284. b
285. a
286. d
287. d
288. c
289. d
290. b
291. b
292. d
293. b
294. d
295. b
296. d
297. b
298. d
299. a
300. d
301. a
302. c
303. b
304. b
305. c
306. d
307. a
308. b
309. b
310. c
311. b
312. d
313. a
314. b
315. a
316. c
317. a
318. c
319. d
320. b
321. c
322. b
323. d
324. d
325. a
326. b
327. c
328. a
329. a
330. c
331. d
332. d
333. a
334. a
335. a
336. c
337. b
338. d
339. c
340. a
341. c
342. c
343. c
344. b
345. a
346. b
347. b
348. a
349. d
350. d
351. a
352. b
353. c
354. b
355. c
356. a
357. a
358. d
359. d
360. a
361. b
362. a
363. c
364. d
365. a
366. d
367. b
368. b
369. d
370. c
371. a
372. b
373. a
374. c
375. c
376. a
377. b
378. b
379. a
380. d
381. a
382. a
383. c
384. a
385. d
386. b
387. b
388. d
389. a
390. b
391. a
392. d
393. b
394. a
395. d
396. c
397. b
398. d
399. a
400. d
401. a
402. b
403. c
404. b
405. d
406. d
407. a
408. b
409. c
410. b
411. c
412. d
413. d
414. a
415. b
416. d
417. c
418. b
419. a
420. a
421. a
422. b
423. c
424. c
425. b
426. a
427. d
428. b
429. d
430. a
431. c
432. c
433. b
434. b
435. a
436. d
437. c
438. c
439. d
440. a
441. d
442. c
443. b
444. a
445. b
446. b
447. c
448. a
449. b
450. a

451. b
452. d
453. a
454. c
455. c
456. c
457. d
458. d
459. a
460. d
461. c
462. c
463. a
464. b
465. a
466. c
467. e
468. d
469. d
470. d
471. b
472. c
473. a
474. c
475. d
476. a
477. b
478. b
479. b
480. c
481. d
482. d
483. a
484. a
485. d
486. b
487. e
488. b
489. d
490. a
491. b
492. a
493. d
494. a
495. a
496. b
497. a
498. c
499. e
500. d
501. d
502. a
503. b
504. d
505. d
506. d
507. a
508. c
509. b
510. a
511. a
512. c
513. b
514. d
515. a
516. b
517. c
518. d
519. a
520. a
521. a
522. d
523. b
524. b
525. d
526. c
527. d
528. b

Titles Available from Silver Educational Publishing

Spinal Anatomy Study Guide: Key Review Questions and Answers

Microbiology Study Guide: Key Review Questions and Answers

Anatomy and Physiology Study Guide: Key Review Questions and Answers with Explanations (Volume 1)

Anatomy and Physiology Study Guide: Key Review Questions and Answers with Explanations (Volume 2)

Key Facts for Anatomy and Physiology

National Board of Chiropractic Part I Study Guide: Key Review Questions and Answers

National Board of Chiropractic Part II Study Guide: Key Review Questions and Answers

National Board of Chiropractic Part III Study Guide: Key Review Questions and Answers with Explanations

The Ultimate Study Guide for the National Certification Examination for Therapeutic Massage and Bodywork: Key Review Questions and Answers
Topics: Human Anatomy, Physiology and Kinesiology (Volume 1)

The Ultimate Study Guide for the National Certification Examination for Therapeutic Massage and Bodywork: Key Review Questions and Answers
Topics: Clinical Pathology & Recognition of Various Conditions (Volume 2)

The Ultimate Study Guide for the National Certification Examination for Therapeutic Massage and Bodywork: Key Review Questions and Answers
Topics: Massage Therapy and Bodywork: Theory, Assessment and Application. Professional Standards, Ethics & Business Practices (Volume 3)